IMG Friendly Anesthesiology Residency Programs List

With Comprehensive Match Selection Criteria and Programs Requirements

By

IMG Guide

And

Applicant Guide

Contents

Introduction

IMG Friendly Anesthesiology Residency Programs List

In Collaboration between the Applicant Guide and the IMG Guide we present to you the most complete and up-to-date IMG friendly anesthesiology residency programs list with full match selection criteria and requirements for these programs. This book is essentially written for international medical graduates seeking residency in the US. The idea of writing this book came from our insight that many IMGs every year don't match because they don't

where to apply. Most of the time, they end
applying to programs that don't have IMGs or
those that don't match their criteria hence they
end losing money with no interviews earned.
The information was gathered from program
directors, coordinators, chiefs, faculty and
residents. It includes Programs names,
Programs codes, States, Addresses, Phones,
Faxes, Percentage of IMGs in the programs,
Minimum USMLE Step 1 and Step 2 Score
Requirements, Attempts on any step, CS
requirement at time of application, USCE
Requirements, Cut-Off time since graduation,
Programs offering couple match and Visas
Sponsored or accepted.

various resources in the residency programs which is/are subject to change by/at the programs at any time. Although we did our best to get the most accurate information as much as possible from the program directors, coordinators, faculty and residents, however, you understand that by reading this book you are using the information here on your own responsibility.

Alabama

University of Alabama Medical Center Anesthesiology Residency Program

Specialty: Anesthesiology
Program name: University of Alabama Medical Center Program
Program code: 040-01-21-010
NRMP Code: 1007040C0
Program type: University-based

State: Alabama
Address: University of Alabama Medical Center, Department of Anesthesiology,
              619 S 19th St, Birmingham, AL 35249-6810
Phone: (205) 934-6525
Fax: (205) 975-0232
Percentage of IMGs in the program: 1%. (Occasionally one IMG)
Minimum USMLE Step 1 Score Requirement: 215
Minimum USMLE Step 2 Score Requirement: No minimum requirement.
Attempts on any step: No strict requirements.
CS required at time of application: No.
USCE Requirement: None.
Cut-Off time since graduation: No limits set.
Program offers couple match: Yes
Visas Sponsored or accepted: H1b visa

Arizona

University of Arizona Anesthesiology Residency Program

Specialty: Anesthesiology
Program name: University of Arizona Program
Program code: 040-03-21-012

NRMP Code: 1015040A0
Program type: University-based
State: Arizona
Address: University of Arizona Health Sciences Center, Anesthesiology Department,
            1501 N Campbell Ave, Tucson, AZ 85724
Phone: (520) 626-7141
Fax: (520) 626-6943
Percentage of IMGs in the program: 5%
Minimum USMLE Step 1 Score Requirement: No minimum requirement.
Minimum USMLE Step 2 Score Requirement: No minimum requirement.
Attempts on any step: No strict requirements.
CS required at time of application: No.
USCE Requirement: None.
Cut-Off time since graduation: No limits set.
Program offers couple match: Yes.
Visas Sponsored or accepted: J1 visa and H1b visa.

Arkansas

University of Arkansas for Medical Sciences Anesthesiology Residency Program

Specialty: Anesthesiology

Program name: University of Arkansas for Medical Sciences Program
Program code: 040-04-21-013
NRMP Code: 1018040C0
Program type: University-based
State: Arkansas
Address: University of Arkansas for Medical Sciences, Department of Anesthesiology, 4301 W Markham St, Slot 515, Little Rock, AR 72205
Phone: (501) 603-1656
Fax: (501) 686-7059
Percentage of IMGs in the program: 32%
Minimum USMLE Step 1 Score Requirement: 205
Minimum USMLE Step 2 Score Requirement: 210
Attempts on any step: 2 maximum attempts, this also apply to the CS exam.
CS required at time of application: No.
USCE Requirement: None.
Cut-Off time since graduation: 5 years.
Program offers couple match: yes.
Visas Sponsored or accepted: J1 visa

California

Loma Linda University Anesthesiology Residency Program

Specialty: Anesthesiology
Program name: Loma Linda University Program
Program code: 040-05-21-016
Program type: University based.
State: California
Address: Loma Linda University Medical Center, Rm 2534, 11234 Anderson St, Loma Linda, CA 92354
Phone: (909) 558-4015
Fax: (909) 558-0214
Percentage of IMGs in the program: 3%
Minimum USMLE Step 1 Score Requirement: No minimum requirement.
Minimum USMLE Step 2 Score Requirement: No minimum requirement.
Attempts on any step: No limits set.
CS required at time of application: Yes, ECFMG certificate as well as PTAL (California letter).
USCE Requirement: None.
Cut-Off time since graduation: No limits set.
Program offers couple match: Yes.
Visas Sponsored or accepted: J1 visa and H1b visa.

UCLA Medical Center
Anesthesiology Residency Program

Specialty: Anesthesiology
Program name: UCLA Medical Center Program
Program code: 040-05-21-020
NRMP Code: 1956040C0
Program type: University-based.
State: California
Address: UCLA Medical Center, Department of Anesthesiology, Suite 3304
757 Westwood Plaza, Los Angeles, CA 90095-7403
Phone: (310) 267-8655
Fax: (310) 267-3766
Percentage of IMGs in the program: 3%
Minimum USMLE Step 1 Score Requirement: 210
Minimum USMLE Step 2 Score Requirement: No minimum requirement.
Attempts on any step: No strict requirements.
CS required at time of application: No, but PTAL required.
USCE Requirement: None.
Cut-Off time since graduation: No limits set.
Program offers couple match: Yes.
Visas Sponsored or accepted: J1 visa

University of Southern California/LAC USC Medical Center Anesthesiology Residency Program

Specialty: Anesthesiology
Program name: University of Southern California/LAC USC Medical Center Program
Program code: 040-05-21-018
State: California
Address: LAC+USC Medical Center, IPT C4E100
2051 Marengo St, Los Angeles, CA 90033
Phone: (323) 409-7748
Fax: (323) 441-8029
Percentage of IMGs in the program: 5%
Minimum USMLE Step 1 Score Requirement: 225
Minimum USMLE Step 2 Score Requirement: 225
Attempts on any step: Must pass from first attempt, this includes CS exam.
CS required at time of application: No, but PTAL status is required.
USCE Requirement: 12 months
Cut-Off time since graduation: No limits set.
Program offers couple match: Yes
Visas Sponsored or accepted: J1 visa

University of California (Davis) Health System Anesthesiology Residency Program

Specialty: Anesthesiology
Program name: University of California (Davis) Health System Program
Program code: 040-05-21-014
State: California
Address: UC Davis Medical Center, PSSB Suite 1200

       4150 V St, Sacramento, CA 95817
Phone: (916) 734-5169
Fax: (916) 734-7980
Percentage of IMGs in the program: 5%
Minimum USMLE Step 1 Score Requirement: 210
Minimum USMLE Step 2 Score Requirement: 210
Attempts on any step: No limits
CS required at time of application: Yes, as well as ECFMG certificate and PTAL.
USCE Requirement: None.
Cut-Off time since graduation: No limits set.
Program offers couple match: Yes.
Visas Sponsored or accepted: No visa

University of California (San Diego) Anesthesiology Residency Program

Specialty: Anesthesiology
Program name: University of California (San Diego) Program
Program code: 040-05-21-022
State: California
Address: UCSD Med Center, MC 8770
200 W Arbor Dr, San Diego, CA 92103-8770
Phone: (619) 543-5297
Fax: (619) 543-6476
Percentage of IMGs in the program: 5%
Minimum USMLE Step 1 Score Requirement: No minimum requirements.
Minimum USMLE Step 2 Score Requirement: No minimum requirements.
Attempts on any step: No strict requirements.
CS required at time of application: Yes as well as the ECFMG certificate and PTAL status.
USCE Requirement: None.
Cut-Off time since graduation: No limits set.
Program offers couple match: Yes
Visas Sponsored or accepted: J1 visa

University of Illinois College of Medicine at Chicago Anesthesiology Residency Program

Specialty: Anesthesiology
Program name: University of Illinois College of Medicine at Chicago Program
Program code: 040-16-11-041
NRMP Code: 1150040C0
Program type: University-based
State: Illinois
Address: University of Illinois Med Center, Suite 3200W M/C 515,
          1740 W Taylor St, Chicago, IL 60612-7239
Phone: (312) 996-4021
Fax: (312) 996-4019
Percentage of IMGs in the program: 3%
Minimum USMLE Step 1 Score Requirement: 220
Minimum USMLE Step 2 Score Requirement: No limits set
Attempts on any step: Must pass first attempt including CS exam
CS required at time of application: No
USCE Requirement: None
Cut-Off time since graduation: 5 years
Program offers couple match: Yes
Visas Sponsored or accepted: J1 visa

University of California (San Francisco) Anesthesiology Residency Program

Specialty: Anesthesiology
Program name: University of California (San Francisco) Program
Program code: 040-05-21-023
State: California
Address: UCSF Medical Center, Rm S436 Box 0427

513 Parnassus Ave San Francisco, CA 94143-0427
Phone: (415) 476-3235
Fax: (415) 514-0185
Percentage of IMGs in the program: 5%
Minimum USMLE Step 1 Score Requirement: 230 for IMGs
Minimum USMLE Step 2 Score Requirement: 230 for IMGs
Attempts on any step: Prefer applicants with no attempts.
CS required at time of application: No
USCE Requirement: Yes, but no specific requirements.
Cut-Off time since graduation: No limits set.
Program offers couple match: Yes
Visas Sponsored or accepted: J1 visa

Cedars-Sinai Medical Center Anesthesiology Residency Program

Specialty: Anesthesiology
Program name: Cedars-Sinai Medical Center Program
Program code: 040-05-21-019
NRMP Code: 1030040C0
Program type: Community-based university affiliated hospital
State: California
Address: Cedars-Sinai Medical Center, Department of Anesthesiology
8700 Beverly Blvd, Los Angeles, CA 90048
Phone: (310) 423-1682
Fax: (310) 423-4119
Percentage of IMGs in the program: 3%
Minimum USMLE Step 1 Score Requirement: 225
Minimum USMLE Step 2 Score Requirement: 225
Attempts on any step: Applicant must pass on first attempt.
CS required at time of application: No
USCE Requirement: None
Cut-Off time since graduation: No limits set
Program offers couple match: Yes
Visas Sponsored or accepted: J1 visa and H1b visa

Stanford University Anesthesiology Residency Program

Specialty: Anesthesiology
Program name: Stanford University Program
Program code: 040-05-21-025
NRMP Code: 1820742C0, 1820040C0
Program type: University-based
State: California
Address: Stanford University Medical Center, Rm H3580

   300 Pasteur Dr, Stanford, CA 94305-5117
Phone: (650) 723-7377
Fax: (650) 725-8544
Percentage of IMGs in the program: 0 - 4% (variable)
Minimum USMLE Step 1 Score Requirement: 210
Minimum USMLE Step 2 Score Requirement: 210
Attempts on any step: Applicant must pass on first attempt
CS required at time of application: Yes, as well as ECFMG certificate and PTAL status.
USCE Requirement: Yes
Cut-Off time since graduation: No limits set
Program offers couple match: Yes
Visas Sponsored or accepted: J1 visa

Los Angeles County-Harbor-UCLA Medical Center Anesthesiology Residency Program

Specialty: Anesthesiology
Program name: Los Angeles County-Harbor-UCLA Medical Center Program
Program code: 040-05-11-026
Program type: Community-based university affiliated hospital
State: California
Address: Los Angeles County-Harbor-UCLA Medical Center, Box 10
          1000 W Carson St, Torrance, CA 90509-2910
Phone: (310) 222-5067
Fax: (310) 222-5252
Percentage of IMGs in the program: 8%
Minimum USMLE Step 1 Score Requirement: 210
Minimum USMLE Step 2 Score Requirement: 210
Attempts on any step: Prefer applicants who passed on their first attempt.
CS required at time of application: Yes as well as the ECFMG certificate and PTAL status.
USCE Requirement: None
Cut-Off time since graduation: No limits set
Program offers couple match: Yes

Visas Sponsored or accepted: No visa

Connecticut

University of Connecticut Anesthesiology Residency Program

Specialty: Anesthesiology
Program name: University of Connecticut Program
Program code: 040-08-21-172
NRMP Code: 1094040C0
Program type: University-based
State: Connecticut
Address: University of Connecticut Health Center, Department of Anesthesiology,
          263 Farmington Ave, Farmington, CT 06030-2015
Phone: (860) 679-3600
Fax: (860) 679-1275
Percentage of IMGs in the program: 30%
Minimum USMLE Step 1 Score Requirement: 205
Minimum USMLE Step 2 Score Requirement: 205
Attempts on any step: No limits set.
CS required at time of application: Yes as well as the ECFMG certificate.
USCE Requirement: None

Cut-Off time since graduation: Within 5 years.
Program offers couple match: Yes
Visas Sponsored or accepted: J1 visa

Yale-New Haven Medical Center Anesthesiology Residency Program

Specialty: Anesthesiology
Program name: Yale-New Haven Medical Center Program
Program code: 040-08-21-030
NRMP Code: 1089040C0
Program type: University-based
State: Connecticut
Address: Yale-New Haven Medical Center, Department of Anesthesiology
20 York St, New Haven, CT 06510
Phone: (203) 737-5165
Fax: (203) 785-6664
Percentage of IMGs in the program: 18%
Minimum USMLE Step 1 Score Requirement: 205
Minimum USMLE Step 2 Score Requirement: 205
Attempts on any step: No limits set
CS required at time of application: Yes as well as ECFMG certificate.
USCE Requirement: Yes
Cut-Off time since graduation: No limits set

Program offers couple match: Yes
Visas Sponsored or accepted: J1 visa

Florida

University of Florida Anesthesiology Residency Program

Specialty: Anesthesiology
Program name: University of Florida Program
Program code: 040-11-21-035
NRMP Code: 1824040C0, 1824040C1
Program type: University-based
State: Florida
Address: University of Florida College of Medicine, PO Box 100254,
               1600 SW Archer Rd, Gainesville, FL 32610-0254
Phone: (352) 594-5766
Fax: (352) 265-6922
Percentage of IMGs in the program: 15%
Minimum USMLE Step 1 Score Requirement: 205
Minimum USMLE Step 2 Score Requirement: 205
Attempts on any step: Must pass first attempt
CS required at time of application: Yes as well as ECFMG certificate.
USCE Requirement: No

Cut-Off time since graduation: No limits set but prefer recent graduates.
Program offers couple match: Yes
Visas Sponsored or accepted: No visa

College of Medicine Mayo Clinic (Jacksonville) Anesthesiology Residency Program

Specialty: Anesthesiology
Program name: Mayo Clinic College of Medicine (Jacksonville) Program
Program code: 040-11-13-194
NRMP Code: 1032040C0
Program type: Community-based university affiliated hospital
State: Florida
Address: Mayo Clinic Jacksonville, Stabile 790N, 4500 San Pablo Rd, Jacksonville, FL 32224
Phone: (904) 953-0487
Fax: (904) 953-0430
Percentage of IMGs in the program: 8%
Minimum USMLE Step 1 Score Requirement: 205
Minimum USMLE Step 2 Score Requirement: 205
Attempts on any step: Must pass from first attempt, this also include the CS exam.

CS required at time of application: Yes as well as ECFMG certificate.
USCE Requirement: None
Cut-Off time since graduation: No limits set
Program offers couple match: Yes
Visas Sponsored or accepted: J1 visa and H1b visa

Jackson Memorial Hospital/Jackson Health System Anesthesiology Residency Program

Specialty: Anesthesiology
Program name: Jackson Memorial Hospital/Jackson Health System Program
Program code: 040-11-21-036
NRMP Code: 1104040C3
Program type: Community-based university affiliated hospital
State: Florida
Address: University of Miami/Jackson Memorial Hospital
        Department of Anesthesiology SW Bldg #303,
        1611 NW 12th Ave, Miami, FL 33136
Phone: (305) 585-6973 Ext: 4
Fax: (305) 585-8359
Percentage of IMGs in the program: 25%

Minimum USMLE Step 1 Score Requirement:
205
Minimum USMLE Step 2 Score Requirement:
205
Attempts on any step: No limits set.
CS required at time of application: Yes as well
as the ECFMG certificate.
USCE Requirement: None.
Cut-Off time since graduation: No limits set
Program offers couple match: Yes
Visas Sponsored or accepted: J1 visa

Georgia

Medical College of Georgia Anesthesiology Residency Program

Specialty: Anesthesiology
Program name: Medical College of Georgia
Program
Program code: 040-12-11-038
NRMP Code: 1985040C0
Program type: University-based
State: Georgia
Address: Georgia Regents University MCG,
Department of Anesthesiology BIW-2144,
1120 15th St, Augusta, GA 30912-2700
Phone: (706) 721-4544

Fax: (706) 721-7753
Percentage of IMGs in the program: 14%
Minimum USMLE Step 1 Score Requirement: 205
Minimum USMLE Step 2 Score Requirement: 205
Attempts on any step: Must pass any step first attempt.
CS required at time of application: No.
USCE Requirement: None.
Cut-Off time since graduation: No limits set.
Program offers couple match: Yes
Visas Sponsored or accepted: J1 visa

Illinois

Advocate Illinois Masonic Medical Center Anesthesiology Residency Program

Specialty: Anesthesiology
Program name: Advocate Illinois Masonic Medical Center Program
Program code: 040-16-21-040
NRMP Code: 1137040C0, 1137040R0
Program type: Community-based university affiliated hospital
State: Illinois

Address: Advocate Illinois Masonic Med Center, Department of Anesthesiology,
836 W Wellington Ave, Chicago, IL 60657-5193
Phone: (773) 296-7035
Fax: (773) 296-5088
Percentage of IMGs in the program: 45%
Minimum USMLE Step 1 Score Requirement: 220
Minimum USMLE Step 2 Score Requirement: 220
Attempts on any step: Maximum of 2 attempts.
CS required at time of application: No
USCE Requirement: Not a strict requirement but preferred.
Cut-Off time since graduation: Not a strict requirement but prefer within 5 years.
Program offers couple match: Yes
Visas Sponsored or accepted: J1 visa

John H Stroger Hospital of Cook County Anesthesiology Residency Program

Specialty: Anesthesiology
Program name: John H Stroger Hospital of Cook County Program
Program code: 040-16-12-039
NRMP Code: 1127040C0

Program type: Community-based university affiliated hospital
State: Illinois
Address: Stroger Hospital of Cook County, Suite 5678

　　　1901 W Harrison St, Chicago, IL 60612-3798
Phone: (312) 864-1903
Fax: (312) 864-9536
Percentage of IMGs in the program: 80%
Minimum USMLE Step 1 Score Requirement: 220
Minimum USMLE Step 2 Score Requirement: 220
Attempts on any step: No limits set.
CS required at time of application: Yes as well as ECFMG certificate.
USCE Requirement: None.
Cut-Off time since graduation: 5 years.
Program offers couple match: No
Visas Sponsored or accepted: J1 visa

Rush University Medical Center Anesthesiology Residency Program

Specialty: Anesthesiology
Program name: Rush University Medical Center Program
Program code: 040-16-21-043
NRMP Code: 1147040C0, 1147040R0

Program type: University-based
State: Illinois
Address: Rush University Medical Center, Department of Anesthesiology,
          1653 W Congress Pkwy, Chicago, IL 60612
Phone: (312) 942-3134
Fax: (312) 942-8858
Percentage of IMGs in the program: 15%
Minimum USMLE Step 1 Score Requirement: 220
Minimum USMLE Step 2 Score Requirement: 220
Attempts on any step: Maximum 2 allowed.
CS required at time of application: Yes as well as ECFMG certificate.
USCE Requirement: None
Cut-Off time since graduation: 5 years
Program offers couple match: Yes
Visas Sponsored or accepted: H1b visa

Loyola University Anesthesiology Residency Program

Specialty: Anesthesiology
Program name: Loyola University Program
Program code: 040-16-11-046
Program type: University-based
State: Illinois
Address: Loyola University Med Center, Department of Anesthesiology,

2160 S First Ave, Maywood, IL 60153
Phone: (708) 216-9169
Fax: (708) 216-1249
Percentage of IMGs in the program: 5%
Minimum USMLE Step 1 Score Requirement: 210
Minimum USMLE Step 2 Score Requirement: 210
Attempts on any step: Must pass first attempt
CS required at time of application: No
USCE Requirement: 6 months
Cut-Off time since graduation: 2 years
Program offers couple match: Yes
Visas Sponsored or accepted: J1 visa

University of Illinois College of Medicine at Chicago Anesthesiology Residency Program

Specialty: Anesthesiology
Program name: University of Illinois College of Medicine at Chicago Program
Program code: 040-16-11-041
NRMP Code: 1150040C0
Program type: University-based
State: Illinois
Address: University of Illinois Med Center, Suite 3200W M/C 515,

1740 W Taylor St, Chicago, IL 60612-7239
Phone: (312) 996-4021
Fax: (312) 996-4019
Percentage of IMGs in the program: 3%
Minimum USMLE Step 1 Score Requirement: 220
Minimum USMLE Step 2 Score Requirement: No limits set
Attempts on any step: Must pass first attempt including CS exam
CS required at time of application: No
USCE Requirement: None
Cut-Off time since graduation: 5 years
Program offers couple match: Yes
Visas Sponsored or accepted: J1 visa

Indiana

Indiana University School of Medicine Anesthesiology Residency Program

Specialty: Anesthesiology
Program name: Indiana University School of Medicine Program
Program code: 040-17-21-048
NRMP Code: 1187040C0

Program type: University-based
State: Indiana
Address: Indiana University School of Medicine, Department of Anesthesia Fesler Hall 204,
1120 South Dr, Indianapolis, IN 46202
Phone: (317) 274-0076
Fax: (317) 274-0256
Percentage of IMGs in the program: 20%
Minimum USMLE Step 1 Score Requirement: 220
Minimum USMLE Step 2 Score Requirement: No limits set
Attempts on any step: No limits set
CS required at time of application: Yes as well as the ECFMG certificate
USCE Requirement: None
Cut-Off time since graduation: No limits set
Program offers couple match: Yes
Visas Sponsored or accepted: J1 visa

Iowa

University of Iowa Hospitals and Clinics Anesthesiology Residency Program

Specialty: Anesthesiology

Program name: University of Iowa Hospitals and Clinics Program
Program code: 040-18-21-049
NRMP Code: 1203040C0
Program type: University-based
State: Iowa
Address: University of Iowa Hospitals and Clinics, Department of Anesthesia,
        200 Hawkins Dr, Iowa City, IA 52242-1009
Phone: (319) 356-4076
Fax: (319) 356-2940
Percentage of IMGs in the program: 7%
Minimum USMLE Step 1 Score Requirement: 220
Minimum USMLE Step 2 Score Requirement: 220
Attempts on any step: Must pass on first attempt including CS exam.
CS required at time of application: Yes including ECFMG certificate.
USCE Requirement: None
Cut-Off time since graduation: 7 years
Program offers couple match: Yes
Visas Sponsored or accepted: J1 visa and H1b visa

Kansas

University of Kansas (Wichita) Anesthesiology Residency Program

Specialty: Anesthesiology

Program name: University of Kansas (Wichita) Program

Program code: 040-19-22-051

NRMP Code: 3054040C0

Program type: Community-based university affiliated hospital

State: Kansas

Address: The University of Kansas School of Medicine-Wichita

Via Christi Regional Medical Center-St. Francis Campus

Department of Anesthesiology, Rm 8074,

929 N St Francis, Wichita, KS 67214-3882

Phone: (316) 268-6147

Fax: (316) 291-7759

Percentage of IMGs in the program: 18%

Minimum USMLE Step 1 Score Requirement: 205

Minimum USMLE Step 2 Score Requirement: 205

Attempts on any step: Maximum of 2 attempts on any step.

CS required at time of application: No

USCE Requirement: Yes

Cut-Off time since graduation: 3 years

Program offers couple match: Yes

Visas Sponsored or accepted: J1 visa

Kentucky

University of Kentucky College of Medicine Anesthesiology Residency Program

Specialty: Anesthesiology
Program name: University of Kentucky College of Medicine Program
Program code: 040-20-21-052
NRMP Code: 1848040C0
Program type: University-based
State: Kentucky
Address: University of Kentucky Med Center, Department of Anesthesiology N253,
800 Rose St, Lexington, KY 40536-0293
Phone: (859) 323-5956   Ext: 80089
Fax: (859) 323-1080
Percentage of IMGs in the program: 5%
Minimum USMLE Step 1 Score Requirement: No limits set
Minimum USMLE Step 2 Score Requirement: No limits set
Attempts on any step: No limits set
CS required at time of application: No
USCE Requirement: None

Cut-Off time since graduation: No limits set
Program offers couple match: Yes
Visas Sponsored or accepted: J1 visa

University of Louisville Anesthesiology Residency Program

Specialty: Anesthesiology
Program name: University of Louisville Program
Program code: 040-20-21-053
NRMP Code: 1217040C0
Program type: University-based
State: Kentucky
Address: University of Louisville Hospital, Department of Anesthesiology
530 S Jackson St, Louisville, KY 40202
Phone: (502) 852-5851
Fax: (502) 852-3762
Percentage of IMGs in the program: 15%
Minimum USMLE Step 1 Score Requirement: No limits set
Minimum USMLE Step 2 Score Requirement: No limits set
Attempts on any step: Must pass first attempt including the CS exam
CS required at time of application: Yes including ECFMG certificate
USCE Requirement: None
Cut-Off time since graduation: No limits set

Program offers couple match: Yes
Visas Sponsored or accepted: J1 visa

Louisiana

Ochsner Clinic Foundation Anesthesiology Residency Program

Specialty: Anesthesiology
Program name: Ochsner Clinic Foundation Program
Program code: 040-21-12-055
NRMP Code: 1966040C0
Program type: Community-based
State: Louisiana
Address: Ochsner Clinic Foundation, Department of Anesthesia,
          1514 Jefferson Hwy,New Orleans, LA 70121
Phone: (504) 842-3755
Percentage of IMGs in the program: 5%
Minimum USMLE Step 1 Score Requirement: 210
Minimum USMLE Step 2 Score Requirement: 210
Attempts on any step: No limits set
CS required at time of application: Yes as well as ECFMG certificate

USCE Requirement: Yes, 12 months.
Cut-Off time since graduation: 5 years
Program offers couple match: Yes
Visas Sponsored or accepted: J1 visa

Tulane University Anesthesiology Residency Program

Specialty: Anesthesiology
Program name: Tulane University Program
Program code: 040-21-31-168
Program type: University-based
State: Louisiana
Address: Tulane University School of Medicine,Anesthesiology SL4,
            1430 Tulane Ave, New Orleans, LA 70112
Phone: (504) 988-5904
Fax: (504) 988-1941
Percentage of IMGs in the program: 5%
Minimum USMLE Step 1 Score Requirement: 230
Minimum USMLE Step 2 Score Requirement: 230
Attempts on any step: Must pass from first attempt on any step including the CS exam.
CS required at time of application: Yes as well as ECFMG certificate
USCE Requirement: Yes, 12 months
Cut-Off time since graduation: 5 years

Program offers couple match: Yes
Visas Sponsored or accepted: No visa

Louisiana State University (Shreveport) Anesthesiology Residency Program

Specialty: Anesthesiology
Program name: Louisiana State University (Shreveport) Program
Program code: 040-21-11-056
Program type: University-based
State: Louisiana
Address: LSU Health Science Center Shreveport, PO Box 33932,
          1501 Kings Hwy, Shreveport, LA 71130-3932
Phone: (318) 675-7195
Fax: (318) 675-4744
Percentage of IMGs in the program: 20%
Minimum USMLE Step 1 Score Requirement: No limits set
Minimum USMLE Step 2 Score Requirement: No limits set
Attempts on any step: No limits set
CS required at time of application: Yes including ECFMG certificate
USCE Requirement: None
Cut-Off time since graduation: No limits set

Program offers couple match: Yes
Visas Sponsored or accepted: J1 visa

Maryland

Johns Hopkins University Anesthesiology Residency Program

Specialty: Anesthesiology
Program name: Johns Hopkins University Program
Program code: 040-23-21-058
Program type: University-based
State: Maryland
Address: Johns Hopkins Hospital, Bloomberg 6220,
          600 N Wolfe St, Baltimore, MD 21287-4963
Phone: (410) 955-7615
Fax: (410) 955-9149
Percentage of IMGs in the program: 5%
Minimum USMLE Step 1 Score Requirement: No limits set
Minimum USMLE Step 2 Score Requirement: No limits set
Attempts on any step: Must pass from first attempt including the CS exam
CS required at time of application: No
USCE Requirement: Yes
Cut-Off time since graduation: No limits set

Program offers couple match: Yes
Visas Sponsored or accepted: J1 visa

Massachusetts

Beth Israel Deaconess Medical Center Anesthesiology Residency Program

Specialty: Anesthesiology
Program name: Beth Israel Deaconess Medical Center Program
Program code: 040-24-11-060
NRMP Code: 1256040C0
Program type: University-based
State: Massachusetts
Address: Beth Israel Deaconess Med Center, Department of Anesthesia CC-470,
          One Deaconess Rd, Boston, MA 02215
Phone: (617) 754-2713
Fax: (617) 754-2735
Percentage of IMGs in the program: 10%
Minimum USMLE Step 1 Score Requirement: 220
Minimum USMLE Step 2 Score Requirement: 220
Attempts on any step: Must pass from first attempt on any step including CS exam
CS required at time of application: Yes including ECFMG certificate

USCE Requirement: None
Cut-Off time since graduation: No limits set
Program offers couple match: Yes
Visas Sponsored or accepted: J1 visa and H1b visa

Boston Medical Center Anesthesiology Residency Program

Specialty: Anesthesiology
Program name: Boston Medical Center Program
Program code: 040-24-21-062
NRMP Code: 1257040C0
Program type: University-based
State: Massachusetts
Address: Boston Medical Center, Department of Anesthesiology Rm 2817,
          88 E Newton St, Boston, MA 02118
Phone: (617) 638-6975
Fax: (617) 638-6959
Percentage of IMGs in the program: 10%
Minimum USMLE Step 1 Score Requirement: 220
Minimum USMLE Step 2 Score Requirement: 220
Attempts on any step: Must pass from first attempt
CS required at time of application: Yes including ECFMG certificate

USCE Requirement: None
Cut-Off time since graduation: No limits set
Program offers couple match: Yes
Visas Sponsored or accepted: No visa

Brigham and Women Hospital Anesthesiology Residency Program

Specialty: Anesthesiology
Program name: Brigham and Women's Hospital Program
Program code: 040-24-21-066
NRMP Code: 1265040C0
Program type: University-based
State: Massachusetts
Address: Brigham and Women's Hospital, Department of Anesthesiology,
           75 Francis St, Boston, MA 02115
Phone: (617) 732-8218
Fax: (617) 582-6131
Percentage of IMGs in the program: 10%
Minimum USMLE Step 1 Score Requirement: No limits set
Minimum USMLE Step 2 Score Requirement: No limits set
Attempts on any step: No limits set
CS required at time of application: No
USCE Requirement: None
Cut-Off time since graduation: No limits set

Program offers couple match: Yes
Visas Sponsored or accepted: J1 visa and H1b visa

St. Elizabeth Medical Center Anesthesiology Residency Program

Specialty: Anesthesiology
Program name: St Elizabeth's Medical Center Program
Program code: 040-24-21-067
State: Massachusetts
Address: St Elizabeth's Medical Center, CMP-2 #213,

736 Cambridge St, Boston, MA 02135-2997
Phone: (617) 789-2777
Fax: (617) 254-6384
Percentage of IMGs in the program: 40%
Minimum USMLE Step 1 Score Requirement: No limits set
Minimum USMLE Step 2 Score Requirement: No limits set
Attempts on any step: No limits set
CS required at time of application: No
USCE Requirement: Yes.
Cut-Off time since graduation: No limits set
Program offers couple match: Yes
Visas Sponsored or accepted: J1 visa

Massachusetts General Hospital Anesthesiology Residency Program

Specialty: Anesthesiology
Program name: Massachusetts General Hospital Program
Program code: 040-24-31-064
State: Massachusetts
Address: Massachusetts General Hospital, Department of Anesthesia GRB444,
            55 Fruit St, Boston, MA 02114
Phone: (617) 726-3030
Fax: (617) 724-8500
Percentage of IMGs in the program: 8%
Minimum USMLE Step 1 Score Requirement: No limits set
Minimum USMLE Step 2 Score Requirement: No limits set
Attempts on any step: Must pass from first attempt
CS required at time of application: No
USCE Requirement: Yes, 1 month at least.
Cut-Off time since graduation: None
Program offers couple match: Yes
Visas Sponsored or accepted: J1 visa and H1b visa

Tufts Medical Center Anesthesiology Residency Program

Specialty: Anesthesiology
Program name: Tufts Medical Center Program
Program code: 040-24-21-065
Program type: University-based
State: Massachusetts
Address: Tufts Med Center, Department of Anesthesia Box 298,
              800 Washington St, Boston, MA 02111
Phone: (617) 636-9303
Fax: (617) 636-8384
Percentage of IMGs in the program: 18%
Minimum USMLE Step 1 Score Requirement: 225
Minimum USMLE Step 2 Score Requirement: 225
Attempts on any step: No limits set
CS required at time of application: Yes as well as ECFMG certificate
USCE Requirement: Yes
Cut-Off time since graduation: None
Program offers couple match: Yes
Visas Sponsored or accepted: J1 visa

Baystate Medical Center/Tufts University School of Medicine Anesthesiology Residency Program

Specialty: Anesthesiology
Program name: Baystate Medical Center/Tufts University School of Medicine Program
Program code: 040-24-12-069
NRMP Code: 1286040C0
Program type: Community-based university affiliated hospital
State: Massachusetts
Address: Baystate Med Center, Department of Anesthesiology,
759 Chestnut St, Springfield, MA 01199
Phone: (413) 794-4326
Fax: (413) 794-5349
Percentage of IMGs in the program: 30%
Minimum USMLE Step 1 Score Requirement: 207
Minimum USMLE Step 2 Score Requirement: 207
Attempts on any step: Maximum of 2 attempts on any step including CS exam.
CS required at time of application: No
USCE Requirement: None
Cut-Off time since graduation: No limits set
Program offers couple match: Yes
Visas Sponsored or accepted: J1 visa

University of Massachusetts Anesthesiology Residency Program

Specialty: Anesthesiology
Program name: University of Massachusetts Program
Program code: 040-24-31-070
NRMP Code: 3050040C0
Program type: University-based
State: Massachusetts
Address: University of Massachusetts Medical School, Department of Anesthesiology,
55 Lake Ave N, Worcester, MA 01655
Phone: (508) 856-3821
Fax: (508) 856-5911
Percentage of IMGs in the program: 32%
Minimum USMLE Step 1 Score Requirement: 220
Minimum USMLE Step 2 Score Requirement: 220
Attempts on any step: Must pass first attempt on any step including CS exam
CS required at time of application: No
USCE Requirement: None
Cut-Off time since graduation: 10 years
Program offers couple match: Yes
Visas Sponsored or accepted: No visa

Michigan

University of Michigan Anesthesiology Residency Program

Specialty: Anesthesiology
Program name: University of Michigan Program
Program code: 040-25-21-071
NRMP Code: 1293040C0, 1293040R0
Program type: University-based
State: Michigan
Address: University of Michigan Health System, 1H247 UH Box 5048,
1500 E Medical Center Dr, Ann Arbor, MI 48109
Phone: (734) 936-4280
Fax: (734) 936-9091
Percentage of IMGs in the program: 0% but may consider IMGs with previous residency
Minimum USMLE Step 1 Score Requirement: 220
Minimum USMLE Step 2 Score Requirement: 220
Attempts on any step: Must pass from any attempt on any step including CS exam
CS required at time of application: No
USCE Requirement: No
Cut-Off time since graduation: None

Program offers couple match: No
Visas Sponsored or accepted: J1 visa

Henry Ford Hospital/Wayne State University Anesthesiology Residency Program

Specialty: Anesthesiology
Program name: Henry Ford Hospital/Wayne State University Program
Program code: 040-25-21-185
NRMP Code: 1300040C0
Program type: Community-based university affiliated hospital
State: Michigan
Address: Henry Ford Hospital, Department of Anesthesiology K4,

2799 W Grand Blvd, Detroit, MI 48202
Phone: (313) 916-8234
Fax: (313) 916-9434
Percentage of IMGs in the program: 35%
Minimum USMLE Step 1 Score Requirement: 205
Minimum USMLE Step 2 Score Requirement: 205
Attempts on any step: No limits set
CS required at time of application: No
USCE Requirement: None
Cut-Off time since graduation: No limits set

Program offers couple match: No
Visas Sponsored or accepted: J1 visa and H1b visa

Detroit Medical Center/Wayne State University Anesthesiology Residency Program

Specialty: Anesthesiology
Program name: Detroit Medical Center/Wayne State University Program
Program code: 040-25-31-073
NRMP Code: 1295040C0
Program type: University-based
State: Michigan
Address: Harper University Hospital, Box 162 Rm 2901
3990 John R St, Detroit, MI 48201
Phone: (313) 745-7233
Fax: (313) 993-3889
Percentage of IMGs in the program: 50%, prefer those with previous residency.
Minimum USMLE Step 1 Score Requirement: 240
Minimum USMLE Step 2 Score Requirement: 240
Attempts on any step: Must pass on first attempt on any step including CS exam
CS required at time of application: No

USCE Requirement: None
Cut-Off time since graduation: Recent graduates unless with previous residency.
Program offers couple match: Yes
Visas Sponsored or accepted: J1 visa

Minnesota

University of Minnesota Anesthesiology Residency Program

Specialty: Anesthesiology
Program name: University of Minnesota Program
Program code: 040-26-31-075
NRMP Code: 1334040C0
Program type: University-based
State: Minnesota
Address: University of Minnesota Med Center, MMC 294,
            420 Delaware St SE, Minneapolis, MN 55455
Phone: (612) 625-4116
Fax: (612) 626-2363
Percentage of IMGs in the program: 16%
Minimum USMLE Step 1 Score Requirement: No limits set
Minimum USMLE Step 2 Score Requirement: No limits set
Attempts on any step: No limits set

CS required at time of application: No
USCE Requirement: Not a strict requirement but preferred
Cut-Off time since graduation: No limits set
Program offers couple match: Yes
Visas Sponsored or accepted: J1 visa

Mississippi

University of Mississippi Medical Center Anesthesiology Residency Program

Specialty: Anesthesiology
Program name: University of Mississippi Medical Center Program
Program code: 040-27-11-077
NRMP Code: 1957040C0
Program type: University-based
State: Mississippi
Address: University of Mississippi Med Center, Department of Anesthesiology,
         2500 N State St, Jackson, MS 39216
Phone: (601) 984-5900   Ext: 5914
Fax: (601) 984-5915
Percentage of IMGs in the program: 10%
Minimum USMLE Step 1 Score Requirement: No limits set

Minimum USMLE Step 2 Score Requirement:
No limits set
Attempts on any step: No limits set
CS required at time of application: No
USCE Requirement: None
Cut-Off time since graduation: No limits set
Program offers couple match: Yes
Visas Sponsored or accepted: J1 visa

Missouri

University of Missouri-Columbia Anesthesiology Residency Program

Specialty: Anesthesiology
Program name: University of Missouri-Columbia Program
Program code: 040-28-11-078
NRMP Code: 1994040C0
Program type: University-based
State: Missouri
Address: University of Missouri Hospitals and Clinics, Anesthesiology DC005 00,
One Hospital Dr, Columbia, MO 65212
Phone: (573) 884-3466
Fax: (573) 882-2226
Percentage of IMGs in the program: 26%

Minimum USMLE Step 1 Score Requirement: 215
Minimum USMLE Step 2 Score Requirement: 215
Attempts on any step: Must pass on first attempt on any step including CS exam
CS required at time of application: No
USCE Requirement: None
Cut-Off time since graduation: 10 years
Program offers couple match: Yes
Visas Sponsored or accepted: No visa

University of Missouri at Kansas City Anesthesiology Residency Program

Specialty: Anesthesiology
Program name: University of Missouri at Kansas City Program
Program code: 040-28-12-080
NRMP Code: 1343040C0
Program type: University-based
State: Missouri
Address: St Luke's Hospital, Department of Med Education,
          4400 Wornall Rd, Kansas City, MO 64111
Phone: (816) 932-5132
Fax: (816) 932-5179

Percentage of IMGs in the program: 30%
Minimum USMLE Step 1 Score Requirement: 215
Minimum USMLE Step 2 Score Requirement: 215
Attempts on any step: Must pass first attempt on any step including CS exam
CS required at time of application: No
USCE Requirement: None
Cut-Off time since graduation: 5 years
Program offers couple match: Yes
Visas Sponsored or accepted: J1 visa

Washington University/B-JH/SLCH Consortium Anesthesiology Residency Program

Specialty: Anesthesiology
Program name: Washington University/B-JH/SLCH Consortium Program
Program code: 040-28-11-081
NRMP Code: 1353040C0, 1353040C1
Program type: University-based
State: Missouri
Address: Washington University/Barnes-Jewish Hospital, Department of Anesthesiology Box 8054

660 S Euclid Ave, St Louis, MO 63110
Phone: (800) 329-5971
Fax: (314) 747-4284
Percentage of IMGs in the program: 10%

Minimum USMLE Step 1 Score Requirement: No limits set
Minimum USMLE Step 2 Score Requirement: No limits set
Attempts on any step: Must pass first attempt including CS exam
CS required at time of application: Yes
USCE Requirement: None
Cut-Off time since graduation: No limits set
Program offers couple match: Yes
Visas Sponsored or accepted: J1 visa

Nebraska

University of Nebraska Medical Center College of Medicine Anesthesiology Residency Program

Specialty: Anesthesiology
Program name: University of Nebraska Medical Center College of Medicine Program
Program code: 040-30-11-082
NRMP Code: 1376040C0
Program type: University-based
State: Nebraska
Address: University of Nebraska Med Center, Anesthesiology Program,

984455 Nebraska Med Center, Omaha, NE 68198-4455
Phone: (402) 559-7405
Fax: (402) 559-7372
Percentage of IMGs in the program: 10%
Minimum USMLE Step 1 Score Requirement: No limits set
Minimum USMLE Step 2 Score Requirement: No limits set
Attempts on any step: Must pass first attempt
CS required at time of application: No
USCE Requirement: None
Cut-Off time since graduation: 5 years except for those with previous residency
Program offers couple match: Yes
Visas Sponsored or accepted: J1 visa and H1b visa

New Jersey

St. Barnabas Medical Center Anesthesiology Residency Program
Specialty: Anesthesiology
Program name: St Barnabas Medical Center Program
Program code: 040-33-12-085
NRMP Code: 1396040C0

Program type: Community-based university affiliated hospital
State: New Jersey
Address: St Barnabas Medical Center, Department of Anesthesiology,
          94 Old Short Hills Rd, Livingston, NJ 07039
Phone: (973) 322-5512
Fax: (973) 322-8165
Percentage of IMGs in the program: 20%
Minimum USMLE Step 1 Score Requirement: No limits set
Minimum USMLE Step 2 Score Requirement: No limits set
Attempts on any step: Must pass first attempt
CS required at time of application: Yes including ECFMG certificate
USCE Requirement: None
Cut-Off time since graduation: 10 years
Program offers couple match: No
Visas Sponsored or accepted: No visa

UMDNJ-Robert Wood Johnson Medical School Anesthesiology Residency Program

Specialty: Anesthesiology
Program name: Rutgers Robert Wood Johnson Medical School Program

Program code: 040-33-21-180
Program type: University-based
State: New Jersey
Address: Rutgers Robert Wood Johnson Medical School,

Department of Anesthesia CAB Suite 3100,

125 Paterson St, New Brunswick, NJ 08901-1977
Phone: (732) 235-6153
Fax: (732) 235-5100
Percentage of IMGs in the program: 10%
Minimum USMLE Step 1 Score Requirement: No limits set
Minimum USMLE Step 2 Score Requirement: No limits set
Attempts on any step: No limits set
CS required at time of application: Yes including ECFMG certificate
USCE Requirement: Yes
Cut-Off time since graduation: No limits set
Program offers couple match: Yes
Visas Sponsored or accepted: J1 visa

UMDNJ-New Jersey Medical School Anesthesiology Residency Program

Specialty: Anesthesiology
Program name: Rutgers New Jersey Medical School Program

Program code: 040-33-21-087
State: New Jersey
Address: Rutgers New Jersey Med School, PO Box 1709 MSB E-538,
            185 S Orange Ave, Newark, NJ 07103
Phone: (973) 972-0470
Fax: (973) 972-0582
Percentage of IMGs in the program: 15%
Minimum USMLE Step 1 Score Requirement: No limits set
Minimum USMLE Step 2 Score Requirement: No limits set
Attempts on any step: No limits set
CS required at time of application: No
USCE Requirement: None
Cut-Off time since graduation: No limits set
Program offers couple match: No
Visas Sponsored or accepted: J1 visa

Mount Sinai School of Medicine (St Joseph Regional Medical Center) Anesthesiology Residency Program

Specialty: Anesthesiology
Program name: Icahn School of Medicine at Mount Sinai (St Joseph's Regional Medical Center) Program

Program code: 040-33-21-089
Program type: Community-based university affiliated hospital
State: New Jersey
Address: St Joseph's Regional Med Center, Anesthesiology Program,
              703 Main St, Paterson, NJ 07503
Phone: (973) 754-2323
Percentage of IMGs in the program: 80%
Minimum USMLE Step 1 Score Requirement: 205
Minimum USMLE Step 2 Score Requirement: 205
Attempts on any step: Must pass first attempt
CS required at time of application: No
USCE Requirement: None
Cut-Off time since graduation: 5 years
Program offers couple match: No
Visas Sponsored or accepted: J1 visa and H1b visa

New Mexico

University of New Mexico Anesthesiology Residency Program
Specialty: Anesthesiology

Program name: University of New Mexico Program
Program code: 040-34-21-183
Program type: University-based
State: New Mexico
Address: University of New Mexico Health Science Center, MSC10 6000,
　　　　　1 University of New Mexico, Albuquerque, NM 87131
Phone: (505) 272-2734
Fax: (505) 272-1300
Percentage of IMGs in the program: 18%
Minimum USMLE Step 1 Score Requirement: No limits set
Minimum USMLE Step 2 Score Requirement: No limits set
Attempts on any step: No limits set
CS required at time of application: No
USCE Requirement: Yes
Cut-Off time since graduation: No limits set
Program offers couple match: Yes
Visas Sponsored or accepted: J1 visa

New York

Albany Medical Center Anesthesiology Residency Program

Specialty: Anesthesiology
Program name: Albany Medical Center Program
Program code: 040-35-21-167
NRMP Code: 1414040C0
Program type: University-based
State: New York
Address: Albany Med Center, Department of Anesthesiology (131),
          47 New Scotland Ave, Albany, NY 12208-3478
Phone: (518) 262-4302
Fax: (518) 262-4736
Percentage of IMGs in the program: 12%
Minimum USMLE Step 1 Score Requirement: 205
Minimum USMLE Step 2 Score Requirement: 205
Attempts on any step: Must pass first attempt
CS required at time of application: Yes including ECFMG certificate
USCE Requirement: None
Cut-Off time since graduation: N o limits set
Program offers couple match: Yes
Visas Sponsored or accepted: J1 visa

Albert Einstein College of Medicine Anesthesiology Residency Program

Specialty: Anesthesiology
Program name: Albert Einstein College of Medicine Program
Program code: 040-35-21-181
Program type: University-based
State: New York
Address: Montefiore Med Center, Department of Anesthesiology,
          111 E 210th St, Bronx, NY 10467
Phone: (718) 920-4383
Fax: (718) 653-2367
Percentage of IMGs in the program: 10%
Minimum USMLE Step 1 Score Requirement: 205
Minimum USMLE Step 2 Score Requirement: 205
Attempts on any step: Must pass first attempt
CS required at time of application: Yes as well as ECFMG certificate
USCE Requirement: Yes
Cut-Off time since graduation: 5 years
Program offers couple match: Yes
Visas Sponsored or accepted: J1 visa and H1b visa

Maimonides Medical Center Anesthesiology Residency Program

Specialty: Anesthesiology
Program name: Maimonides Medical Center Program
Program code: 040-35-11-101
State: New York
Address: Maimonides Med Center, Anesthesiology Program Office,
931 48th St, Brooklyn, NY 11219
Phone: (718) 283-7176
Fax: (718) 635-7492
Percentage of IMGs in the program: 15%
Minimum USMLE Step 1 Score Requirement: 205
Minimum USMLE Step 2 Score Requirement: 205
Attempts on any step: No limits set
CS required at time of application: No
USCE Requirement: Yes
Cut-Off time since graduation: No limits set
Program offers couple match: Yes
Visas Sponsored or accepted: J1 visa and H1b visa

New York Methodist Hospital Anesthesiology Residency Program

Specialty: Anesthesiology

Program name: New York Methodist Hospital Program
Program code: 040-35-11-102
State: New York
Address: New York Methodist Hospital, Department of Anesthesiology 3rd Fl Carrington Pavilion,
  506 Sixth St, Brooklyn, NY 11215
Phone: (718) 780-3970
Fax: (718) 780-3281
Percentage of IMGs in the program: 85%
Minimum USMLE Step 1 Score Requirement: 210
Minimum USMLE Step 2 Score Requirement: 210
Attempts on any step: Must pass first attempt
CS required at time of application: Yes including ECFMG certificate
USCE Requirement: None
Cut-Off time since graduation: No limits set
Program offers couple match: Yes
Visas Sponsored or accepted: J1 visa and H1b visa

SUNY Health Science Center at Brooklyn Anesthesiology Residency Program

Specialty: Anesthesiology

Program name: SUNY Health Science Center at Brooklyn Program
Program code: 040-35-21-110
NRMP Code: 1426040C0
Program type: University-based
State: New York
Address: SUNY Downstate Med Center, Box 6, 450 Clarkson Ave, Brooklyn, NY 11203
Phone: (718) 270-1926
Fax: (718) 270-3977
Percentage of IMGs in the program: 25%
Minimum USMLE Step 1 Score Requirement: 205
Minimum USMLE Step 2 Score Requirement: 205
Attempts on any step: Must pass on first attempt including CS exam
CS required at time of application: No
USCE Requirement: No
Cut-Off time since graduation: 5 years
Program offers couple match: Yes
Visas Sponsored or accepted: J1 visa

University at Buffalo Anesthesiology Residency Program

Specialty: Anesthesiology
Program name: University at Buffalo Program
Program code: 040-35-21-093

Program type: University-based
State: New York
Address: University at Buffalo School of Med, Department of Anesthesiology,
      252 Farber Hall, Buffalo, NY 14214
Phone: (716) 829-6102
Fax: (716) 829-3640
Percentage of IMGs in the program: 50%
Minimum USMLE Step 1 Score Requirement: 210
Minimum USMLE Step 2 Score Requirement: 210
Attempts on any step: Must pass first attempt including CS exam
CS required at time of application: No
USCE Requirement: None
Cut-Off time since graduation: 2 years
Program offers couple match: Yes
Visas Sponsored or accepted: J1 visa

New York Presbyterian Hospital (Columbia Campus) Anesthesiology Residency Program

Specialty: Anesthesiology
Program name: New York Presbyterian Hospital (Columbia Campus) Program
Program code: 040-35-11-107
State: New York
Address: New York Presbyterian Hospital-Columbia, PH5-133,

622 W 168th St, New York, NY 10032
Phone: (212) 342-5525
Fax: (212) 305-3204
Percentage of IMGs in the program: 20%
Minimum USMLE Step 1 Score Requirement:
210
Minimum USMLE Step 2 Score Requirement:
210
Attempts on any step: No limits set
CS required at time of application: Yes
including ECFMG certificate
USCE Requirement: None
Cut-Off time since graduation: No limits set
Program offers couple match: Yes
Visas Sponsored or accepted: J1 visa

New York Presbyterian Hospital (Cornell Campus) Anesthesiology Residency Program

Specialty: Anesthesiology
Program name: New York Presbyterian Hospital
(Cornell Campus) Program
Program code: 040-35-21-098
NRMP Code: 1492040C0, 1492040R0
Program type: University-based
State: New York
Address: New York Presbyterian Hospital-Weill,
Box 124

525 E 68th St, New York, NY 10065
Phone: (212) 746-2941
Fax: (212) 746-8713
Percentage of IMGs in the program: 10%
Minimum USMLE Step 1 Score Requirement:
No limits set
Minimum USMLE Step 2 Score Requirement:
No limits set
Attempts on any step: No limits set
CS required at time of application: No
USCE Requirement: Not strict but preferred to
have few months.
Cut-Off time since graduation: No limits set
Program offers couple match: Yes
Visas Sponsored or accepted: J1 visa

New York University School of Medicine Anesthesiology Residency Program

Specialty: Anesthesiology
Program name: New York University School of
Medicine Program
Program code: 040-35-21-106
Program type: University-based
State: New York
Address: New York University Med Center,
Department of Anesthesiology Tisch 530,
550 First Ave, New York, NY 10016

Phone: (212) 263-3894
Fax: (212) 263-7254
Percentage of IMGs in the program: 8%
Minimum USMLE Step 1 Score Requirement: No limits set
Minimum USMLE Step 2 Score Requirement: No limits set
Attempts on any step: No limits set
CS required at time of application: No
USCE Requirement: Yes
Cut-Off time since graduation: No limits set
Program offers couple match: Yes
Visas Sponsored or accepted: J1 visa and H1b visa

St. Luke's-Roosevelt Hospital Center Anesthesiology Residency Program

Specialty: Anesthesiology
Program name: St Luke's-Roosevelt Hospital Center Program
Program code: 040-35-11-108
NRMP Code: 2070040C0
Program type: Community-based university affiliated hospital
State: New York
Address: St Luke's-Roosevelt Hospital Center, Department of Anesthesiology,

1111 Amsterdam Ave, New York, NY 10025
Phone: (212) 523-3975
Fax: (212) 523-2602
Percentage of IMGs in the program: 15%
Minimum USMLE Step 1 Score Requirement: No limits set
Minimum USMLE Step 2 Score Requirement: No limits set
Attempts on any step: Must pass first attempt
CS required at time of application: Yes
USCE Requirement: None
Cut-Off time since graduation: No limits set
Program offers couple match: Yes
Visas Sponsored or accepted: J1 visa and H1b visa

University of Rochester Anesthesiology Residency Program

Specialty: Anesthesiology
Program name: University of Rochester Program
Program code: 040-35-11-111
NRMP Code: 1511040C0
Program type: University-based
State: New York
Address: University of Rochester Med Center, Department of Anesthesiology Box 604,

601 Elmwood Ave, Rochester, NY 14642
Phone: (585) 275-1384
Fax: (585) 276-0122
Percentage of IMGs in the program: 18%
Minimum USMLE Step 1 Score Requirement: 205
Minimum USMLE Step 2 Score Requirement: 205
Attempts on any step: Must pass first attempt
CS required at time of application: No
USCE Requirement: None
Cut-Off time since graduation: 10 years
Program offers couple match: Yes
Visas Sponsored or accepted: J1 visa

SUNY at Stony Brook Anesthesiology Residency Program

Specialty: Anesthesiology
Program name: SUNY at Stony Brook Program
Program code: 040-35-21-170
State: New York
Address: SUNY Stony Brook University, Department of Anesthesiology.
HSC L-4 060, Stony Brook, NY 11794
Phone: (631) 444-2975
Fax: (631) 444-2907
Percentage of IMGs in the program: 10%

Minimum USMLE Step 1 Score Requirement:
220
Minimum USMLE Step 2 Score Requirement:
220
Attempts on any step: No limits set
CS required at time of application: Yes as well as ECFMG certificate
USCE Requirement: None
Cut-Off time since graduation: 2 years
Program offers couple match: Yes
Visas Sponsored or accepted: No visa

SUNY Upstate Medical University Anesthesiology Residency Program

Specialty: Anesthesiology
Program name: SUNY Upstate Medical University Program
Program code: 040-35-21-113
NRMP Code: 1516040C0
Program type: University-based
State: New York
Address: SUNY Upstate Med University, Department of Anesthesiology
750 E Adams St, Syracuse, NY 13210
Phone: (315) 464-4889
Fax: (315) 464-4866
Percentage of IMGs in the program: 60%

Minimum USMLE Step 1 Score Requirement:
210
Minimum USMLE Step 2 Score Requirement:
210
Attempts on any step: Must pass first attempt
CS required at time of application: No
USCE Requirement: Yes
Cut-Off time since graduation: 5 years
Program offers couple match: Yes
Visas Sponsored or accepted: J1 visa

New York Medical College at Westchester Medical Center Anesthesiology Residency Program

Specialty: Anesthesiology
Program name: New York Medical College at Westchester Medical Center Program
Program code: 040-35-21-105
Program type: University-based
State: New York
Address: NYMC Westchester Medical Center, Department of Anesthesiology,
Macy Pavilion West Rm 2391, Valhalla, NY 10595
Phone: (914) 493-7692
Fax: (914) 493-7927
Percentage of IMGs in the program: 35%

Minimum USMLE Step 1 Score Requirement: 215
Minimum USMLE Step 2 Score Requirement: 215
Attempts on any step: No limits set
CS required at time of application: No
USCE Requirement: None
Cut-Off time since graduation: No limits set
Program offers couple match: Yes
Visas Sponsored or accepted: J1 visa

Ohio

University Hospital/University of Cincinnati College of Medicine Anesthesiology Residency Program

Specialty: Anesthesiology
Program name: University of Cincinnati Medical Center/College of Medicine Program
Program code: 040-38-21-118
NRMP Code: 1548040C0
Program type: University-based
State: Ohio
Address: University Hospital University of Cincinnati, PO Box 670531,
              231 Albert Sabin Way, Cincinnati, OH 45267

Phone: (513) 558-6356
Fax: (513) 558-0995
Percentage of IMGs in the program: 8%
Minimum USMLE Step 1 Score Requirement: No limits set
Minimum USMLE Step 2 Score Requirement: No limits set
Attempts on any step: No limits set
CS required at time of application: Yes as well as the ECFMG certificate
USCE Requirement: None
Cut-Off time since graduation: No limits set
Program offers couple match: Yes
Visas Sponsored or accepted: J1 visa

Case Western Reserve University (MetroHealth) Anesthesiology Residency Program

Specialty: Anesthesiology
Program name: Case Western Reserve University (MetroHealth) Program
Program code: 040-38-21-174
Program type: University-based
State: Ohio
Address: MetroHealth Med Center, Anesthesiology Program,
        2500 MetroHealth Dr, Cleveland, OH 44109-1998

Phone: (216) 778-3618
Fax: (216) 778-5378
Percentage of IMGs in the program: 25%
Minimum USMLE Step 1 Score Requirement: No limits set
Minimum USMLE Step 2 Score Requirement: No limits set
Attempts on any step: No limits set
CS required at time of application: No
USCE Requirement: Yes, 1 month.
Cut-Off time since graduation: No limits set
Program offers couple match: Yes
Visas Sponsored or accepted: J1 visa and H1b visa

Case Western Reserve University/University Hospitals Case Medical Center Anesthesiology Residency Program

Specialty: Anesthesiology
Program name: Case Western Reserve University/University Hospitals Case Medical Center Program
Program code: 040-38-21-119
State: Ohio
Address: University Hospitals Case Med Center, Department of Anesthesiology& Peri-op Medicine,

11100 Euclid Ave, Cleveland, OH 44106-5007
Phone: (216) 844-7335
Fax: (216) 844-3781
Percentage of IMGs in the program: 0%
Minimum USMLE Step 1 Score Requirement: 210
Minimum USMLE Step 2 Score Requirement: 210
Attempts on any step: No limits set
CS required at time of application: Yes as well as ECFMG certificate
USCE Requirement: None
Cut-Off time since graduation: No limits set
Program offers couple match: Yes
Visas Sponsored or accepted: J1 visa

Ohio State University Hospital Anesthesiology Residency Program

Specialty: Anesthesiology
Program name: Ohio State University Hospital Program
Program code: 040-38-11-123
NRMP Code: 1566040C0
Program type: University-based
State: Ohio
Address: Ohio State University Med Center, N 411 Doan Hall,

410 W 10th Ave, Columbus, OH 43210-1228
Phone: (614) 293-8487
Fax: (614) 293-1578
Percentage of IMGs in the program: 8%
Minimum USMLE Step 1 Score Requirement: No limits set
Minimum USMLE Step 2 Score Requirement: No limits set
Attempts on any step: No limits set
CS required at time of application: Yes including the ECFMG certificate
USCE Requirement: Yes
Cut-Off time since graduation: No limits set
Program offers couple match: Yes
Visas Sponsored or accepted: J1 visa

University of Toledo Anesthesiology Residency Program

Specialty: Anesthesiology
Program name: University of Toledo Program
Program code: 040-38-21-125
State: Ohio
Address: University of Toledo Med Center, Department of Anesthesiology Mail Stop 1137, 3000 Arlington Ave, Toledo, OH 43614
Phone: (419) 383-3507
Fax: (419) 383-3550

Percentage of IMGs in the program: 50%
Minimum USMLE Step 1 Score Requirement: 205
Minimum USMLE Step 2 Score Requirement: 205
Attempts on any step: Must pass from first attempt
CS required at time of application: No
USCE Requirement: None
Cut-Off time since graduation: 5 years
Program offers couple match: Yes
Visas Sponsored or accepted: J1 visa

Cleveland Clinic Foundation Anesthesiology Residency Program

Specialty: Anesthesiology
Program name: Cleveland Clinic Foundation Program
Program code: 040-38-22-120
NRMP Code: 1968040C0
Program type: Community-based
State: Ohio
Address: Cleveland Clinic, Anesthesiology Inst E30,
9500 Euclid Ave, Cleveland, OH 44195
Phone: (216) 445-2115
Fax: (216) 445-0605
Percentage of IMGs in the program: 30%

Minimum USMLE Step 1 Score Requirement:
No limits set
Minimum USMLE Step 2 Score Requirement:
No limits set
Attempts on any step: No limits set
CS required at time of application: Yes
including the ECFMG certificate
USCE Requirement: None
Cut-Off time since graduation: No limits set
Program offers couple match: Yes
Visas Sponsored or accepted: J1 visa and H1b
visa

Oklahoma

University of Oklahoma Health Sciences Center Anesthesiology Residency Program

Specialty: Anesthesiology
Program name: University of Oklahoma Health
Sciences Center Program
Program code: 040-39-21-128
NRMP Code: 1588040C0
Program type: University-based
State: Oklahoma

Address: University of Oklahoma Health Sciences Center, Department of Anesthesiology Suite 200,

750 NE 13th St, Oklahoma City, OK 73104

Phone: (405) 271-4351 Ext: 55019

Fax: (405) 271-8695

Percentage of IMGs in the program: 4%

Minimum USMLE Step 1 Score Requirement: 210

Minimum USMLE Step 2 Score Requirement: 210

Attempts on any step: Must pass on first attempt.

CS required at time of application: Yes as well as the ECFMG certificate.

USCE Requirement: None but preferred.

Cut-Off time since graduation: 2 years

Program offers couple match: Yes

Visas Sponsored or accepted: J1 visa

Pennsylvania

Penn State University/Milton S Hershey Medical Center Anesthesiology Residency Program

Specialty: Anesthesiology

Program name: Penn State Milton S Hershey Medical Center Program

Program code: 040-41-11-130
NRMP Code: 1617040C0
Program type: University-based
State: Pennsylvania
Address: Milton S Hershey Med Center,
Department of Anesthesiology H187,
        500 University Dr, Hershey, PA 17033
Phone: (800) 206-7718
Fax: (717) 531-0826
Percentage of IMGs in the program: 20%
Minimum USMLE Step 1 Score Requirement:
210
Minimum USMLE Step 2 Score Requirement:
210
Attempts on any step: No limits set
CS required at time of application: No
USCE Requirement: None
Cut-Off time since graduation: 5 years
Program offers couple match: Yes
Visas Sponsored or accepted: J1 visa

Drexel University College of Medicine/Hahnemann University Hospital Anesthesiology Residency Program

Specialty: Anesthesiology

Program name: Drexel University College of Medicine/Hahnemann University Hospital Program
Program code: 040-41-21-133
NRMP Code: 1849040C0
Program type: University-based
State: Pennsylvania
Address: Hahnemann University Hospital, MS #310,
          245 N 15th St, Philadelphia, PA 19102-1192
Phone: (215) 762-7922
Fax: (215) 762-8656
Percentage of IMGs in the program: 4%
Minimum USMLE Step 1 Score Requirement: No limits set
Minimum USMLE Step 2 Score Requirement: No limits set
Attempts on any step: Must pass first attempt
CS required at time of application: No
USCE Requirement: None
Cut-Off time since graduation: No limits set
Program offers couple match: Yes
Visas Sponsored or accepted: J1 visa

Temple University Hospital Anesthesiology Residency Program

Specialty: Anesthesiology

Program name: Temple University Hospital Program
Program code: 040-41-31-136
Program type: University-based
State: Pennsylvania
Address: Temple University Hospital, 502-00,
          3401 N Broad St, Philadelphia, PA
19140
Phone: (215) 707-3326
Fax: (215) 707-8028
Percentage of IMGs in the program: 8%
Minimum USMLE Step 1 Score Requirement:
No limits set
Minimum USMLE Step 2 Score Requirement:
No limits set
Attempts on any step: Must pass within 3
attempts
CS required at time of application: Yes
including ECFMG certificate
USCE Requirement: None
Cut-Off time since graduation: No limits set
Program offers couple match: Yes
Visas Sponsored or accepted: J1 visa and H1b
visa

Thomas Jefferson University Anesthesiology Residency Program

Specialty: Anesthesiology

Program name: Thomas Jefferson University Program
Program code: 040-41-21-137
NRMP Code: 1630040C0
Program type: University-based
State: Pennsylvania
Address: Thomas Jefferson University Hospital, Department of Anesthesiology Suite 8290 Gibbon,
111 S 11th St, Philadelphia, PA 19107
Phone: (215) 955-2370
Fax: (215) 955-0677
Percentage of IMGs in the program: 10%
Minimum USMLE Step 1 Score Requirement: 210
Minimum USMLE Step 2 Score Requirement: 210
Attempts on any step: No limits set
CS required at time of application: No
USCE Requirement: None
Cut-Off time since graduation: 3 years
Program offers couple match: Yes
Visas Sponsored or accepted: J1 visa and H1b visa

UPMC Medical Education Anesthesiology Residency Program

Specialty: Anesthesiology
Program name: UPMC Medical Education Program

Program code: 040-41-21-139
NRMP Code: 1652040C0
Program type: University-based
State: Pennsylvania
Address: University of Pittsburgh Med Center, Department of Anesthesiology Suite 910
        3471 Fifth Ave, Pittsburgh, PA 15213
Phone: (412) 692-4506
Fax: (412) 692-4515
Percentage of IMGs in the program: 5%
Minimum USMLE Step 1 Score Requirement: 220
Minimum USMLE Step 2 Score Requirement: 220
Attempts on any step: Must pass first attempt
CS required at time of application: No
USCE Requirement: Yes
Cut-Off time since graduation: No limits set
Program offers couple match: Yes
Visas Sponsored or accepted: J1 visa and H1b visa

Allegheny General Hospital-Western Pennsylvania Hospital Medical Education Consortium (WPH) Anesthesiology Residency Program

Specialty: Anesthesiology
Program name: Allegheny General Hospital-Western Pennsylvania Hospital Medical Education Consortium (WPH) Program
Program code: 040-41-32-141
Program type: Community-based university affiliated hospital
State: Pennsylvania
Address: AGH-WPH Med Education Consortium, Anesthesiology Department,
320 E North Ave, Pittsburgh, PA 15212
Phone: (412) 359-6726
Fax: (412) 359-3483
Percentage of IMGs in the program: 3%
Minimum USMLE Step 1 Score Requirement: No limits set
Minimum USMLE Step 2 Score Requirement: No limits set
Attempts on any step: No limits set
CS required at time of application: No
USCE Requirement: None
Cut-Off time since graduation: No limits set
Program offers couple match: Yes
Visas Sponsored or accepted: J1 visa

Geisinger Health System Anesthesiology Residency Program

Specialty: Anesthesiology
Program name: Geisinger Health System Program
Program code: 040-41-00-205
NRMP Code: 1608040C0, 160804R0
Program type: Community-based
State: Pennsylvania
Address: Geisinger Health System, Anesthesiology Program,
100 N Academy Ave, Danville, PA 17822-2025
Phone: (570) 271-6775
Fax: (570) 271-6762
Percentage of IMGs in the program: 18%
Minimum USMLE Step 1 Score Requirement: 188
Minimum USMLE Step 2 Score Requirement: 203
Attempts on any step: No limits set
CS required at time of application: Yes as well as ECFMG certificate.
USCE Requirement: No
Cut-Off time since graduation: 5 years
Program offers couple match: Yes
Visas Sponsored or accepted: J1 visa and H1b visa

Texas

Texas Tech University Health Sciences Center Paul L Foster School of Medicine Anesthesiology Residency Program

Specialty: Anesthesiology
Program name: Texas Tech University Health Sciences Center Paul L Foster School of Medicine Program
Program code: 040-48-31-203
State: Texas
Address: Texas Tech University Health Science Center- Paul L. Foster School of Medicine, Department of Anesthesiology, 4800 Alberta Ave, El Paso, TX 79905
Phone: 915-545-6560
Fax: 915-545-6984
Percentage of IMGs in the program: 25%
Minimum USMLE Step 1 Score Requirement: No limits set
Minimum USMLE Step 2 Score Requirement: No limits set
Attempts on any step: Maximum of 3 attempts on each component
CS required at time of application: Yes

USCE Requirement: No
Cut-Off time since graduation: No limits set
Program offers couple match: Yes
Visas Sponsored or accepted: J1 visa

Texas Tech University (Lubbock) Anesthesiology Residency Program

Specialty: Anesthesiology
Program name: Texas Tech University (Lubbock) Program
Program code: 040-48-11-153
State: Texas
Address: Texas Tech University HSC Lubbock, Rm 1B350D,
        3601 4th St, Lubbock, TX 79430
Phone: (806) 743-2981 Ext: 225
Fax: (806) 743-2984
Percentage of IMGs in the program: 30%
Minimum USMLE Step 1 Score Requirement: No limits set
Minimum USMLE Step 2 Score Requirement: No limits set
Attempts on any step: Maximum of 2 attempts
CS required at time of application: No
USCE Requirement: None
Cut-Off time since graduation: No limits set
Program offers couple match: Yes
Visas Sponsored or accepted: J1 visa

University of Texas at Houston Anesthesiology Residency Program

Specialty: Anesthesiology
Program name: University of Texas at Houston Program
Program code: 040-48-31-152
NRMP Code: 2923040C0
Program type: Community-based university affiliated hospital
State: Texas
Address: University of Texas Medical School Houston, Suite 5196,
          6431 Fannin St, Houston, TX 77030
Phone: (713) 500-6223
Fax: (713) 500-6270
Percentage of IMGs in the program: 10%
Minimum USMLE Step 1 Score Requirement: 220
Minimum USMLE Step 2 Score Requirement: 220
Attempts on any step: Must pass first attempt including the CS exam
CS required at time of application: Yes including the ECFMG certificate
USCE Requirement: None
Cut-Off time since graduation: 5 years
Program offers couple match: Yes
Visas Sponsored or accepted: No visa

Baylor College of Medicine Anesthesiology Residency Program

Specialty: Anesthesiology
Program name: Baylor College of Medicine Program
Program code: 040-48-31-150
State: Texas
Address: Baylor College of Medicine, Baylor Faculty Center (MS:BCM 120) Suite 1700,
        1709 Dryden Rd, Houston, TX 77030
Phone: (713) 798-5117
Fax: (713) 798-6374
Percentage of IMGs in the program: 10%
Minimum USMLE Step 1 Score Requirement: 220
Minimum USMLE Step 2 Score Requirement: No limits set
Attempts on any step: Must pass any step on first attempt including CS exam
CS required at time of application: No
USCE Requirement: None
Cut-Off time since graduation: No limits set
Program offers couple match: Yes
Visas Sponsored or accepted: J1 visa

University of Texas Southwestern Medical School Anesthesiology Residency Program

Specialty: Anesthesiology

Program name: University of Texas Southwestern Medical School Program
Program code: 040-48-21-147
NRMP Code: 2835040C0
Program type: Community-based university affiliated hospital
State: Texas
Address: University of Texas Southwestern Med Center, Department of Anesthesiology
        5323 Harry Hines Blvd, Dallas, TX 75390-9068
Phone: (214) 648-4831
Fax: (214) 648-7660
Percentage of IMGs in the program: 4%
Minimum USMLE Step 1 Score Requirement: No limits set
Minimum USMLE Step 2 Score Requirement: No limits set
Attempts on any step: Must pass on first attempt
CS required at time of application: No
USCE Requirement: No
Cut-Off time since graduation: No limits set
Program offers couple match: Yes
Visas Sponsored or accepted: No visa

Vermont

University of Vermont/Fletcher Allen Health Care Anesthesiology Residency Program

Specialty: Anesthesiology
Program name: University of Vermont/Fletcher Allen Health Care Program
Program code: 040-50-11-158
State: Vermont
Address: University of Vermont FAHC, Department of Anesthesiology,
            111 Colchester Ave, Burlington, VT 05401
Phone: (802) 847-2415
Fax: (802) 847-5324
Percentage of IMGs in the program: 4%
Minimum USMLE Step 1 Score Requirement: No limits set
Minimum USMLE Step 2 Score Requirement: No limits set
Attempts on any step: No limits set
CS required at time of application: Yes including the ECFMG certificate
USCE Requirement: None
Cut-Off time since graduation: 2years
Program offers couple match: Yes
Visas Sponsored or accepted: J1 visa

Virginia

Virginia Commonwealth University Health System Anesthesiology Residency Program

Specialty: Anesthesiology
Program name: Virginia Commonwealth University Health System Program
Program code: 040-51-11-160
NRMP Code: 1743040C0
Program type: University-based
State: Virginia
Address: Virginia Commonwealth University Health System, PO Box 980459
1200 E Broad St, Richmond, VA 23298
Phone: (804) 828-0733
Fax: (804) 828-8300
Percentage of IMGs in the program: 5%
Minimum USMLE Step 1 Score Requirement: 225
Minimum USMLE Step 2 Score Requirement: 225
Attempts on any step: Must pass on first attempt including CS exam
CS required at time of application: Yes including ECFMG certificate
USCE Requirement: None
Cut-Off time since graduation: 4 years
Program offers couple match: Yes
Visas Sponsored or accepted: J1 visa

Washington

University of Washington Anesthesiology Residency Program

Specialty: Anesthesiology
Program name: University of Washington Program
Program code: 040-54-21-161
NRMP Code: 1918040C1, 1918040C0, 1918040C2
Program type: University-based
State: Washington
Address: University of Washington School of Medicine, Box 356540,
          1959 NE Pacific St, Seattle, WA 98195-6540
Phone: (206) 543-2773
Fax: (206) 543-2958
Percentage of IMGs in the program: 3%
Minimum USMLE Step 1 Score Requirement: 210
Minimum USMLE Step 2 Score Requirement: 210
Attempts on any step: Must pass first attempt
CS required at time of application: No
USCE Requirement: Yes
Cut-Off time since graduation: No limits set
Program offers couple match: Yes
Visas Sponsored or accepted: J1 visa and H1b visa

West Virginia

West Virginia University Anesthesiology Residency Program

Specialty: Anesthesiology
Program name: West Virginia University Program
Program code: 040-55-11-163
NRMP Code: 1837040C0
Program type: University-based
State: West Virginia
Address: West Virginia University Hospitals, Department of Anesthesiology,
One Medical Center Dr, Morgantown, WV 26506-8255
Phone: (304) 598-4480
Fax: (304) 598-4930
Percentage of IMGs in the program: 8%
Minimum USMLE Step 1 Score Requirement: 225
Minimum USMLE Step 2 Score Requirement: 225
Attempts on any step: Must pass on first attempt
CS required at time of application: Yes including ECFMG Certificate
USCE Requirement: None

Cut-Off time since graduation: No limits set
Program offers couple match: Yes
Visas Sponsored or accepted: J1 visa

Wisconsin

Medical College of Wisconsin Affiliated Hospitals Anesthesiology Residency Program

Specialty: Anesthesiology
Program name: Medical College of Wisconsin Affiliated Hospitals Program
Program code: 040-56-21-165
NRMP Code: 1784040C0
Program type: Community-based university affiliated hospital
State: Wisconsin
Address: Froedtert Memorial Lutheran Hospital, Department of Anesthesiology,
                9200 W Wisconsin Ave, Milwaukee, WI 53226
Phone: (414) 805-6104
Fax: (414) 805-5915
Percentage of IMGs in the program: 25%
Minimum USMLE Step 1 Score Requirement: 235

Minimum USMLE Step 2 Score Requirement: 235
Attempts on any step: Must pass first attempt
CS required at time of application: Yes including ECFMG certificate
USCE Requirement: None
Cut-Off time since graduation: 3 years, unless in previous residency.
Program offers couple match: No
Visas Sponsored or accepted: J1 visa and H1b visa

Please take 1 minute to write and rate our book on Amazon. We wish you a successful match. Thank you for buying our book.

If you have any questions please email us at applicantguide@yahoo.com

IMG Guide
&
Applicant Guide

www.imgguide.com
www.applicantguide.com